MARK LEWIS

Loving Life on a Bike

A Beginner's Guide to Adventure Cycling

Contents

Acknowledgement   iv

1   Chapter 1   1

2   Chapter 2   5

3   Chapter 3   8

4   Chapter 4   18

5   Chapter 5   26

About the Author   31

Acknowledgement

I am so grateful for the very blessed life I have experienced and enjoy. I firmly believe there is a power for good in this Universe, and I have learned how to tap into that Force of Divine Love. In so being, I have attracted some amazing people and programs into my life. First and foremost, I want to give special thanks to PSI Seminars for their guidance and direction in my personal growth work over the last twenty-five years, and Mile Hi Church, with the Centers for Spiritual Living, for my Spiritual growth work and journey. I fully believe that these incredible organizations have been the causal agent for all the good in my life.

There have been so many people in my life that have demonstrated patience, unconditional giving, kindness, and guidance over the years that it would be difficult to name them all. However, I want to extend a very special thank you to Kathy and Cody Waite with Waite Endurance for all the incredible Physical Fitness Coaching they provided. Thank you Kathy Zawadzki, owner of Fast Lab in Centennial, CO, for your cycling coaching and wealth of knowledge. Thank you Dr. Rick and Christine Zimmerman for providing the most amazing place to live and ride my bikes in Morrison, CO. Thank you Michele Lewis for your inspiration and unconditional love during our time together. Thank you Ryan Van Duzer, for your incredible YouTube channel and all the inspiration you share to just "Get Out There." Thank you Diane Haupt for your inspiration and guidance before, during and after my bike tour across the country. Most importantly though, I want to give a heartfelt thank you to my father, Richard Lewis, for his unconditional love allowing me to create the life of my dreams. Without all their support, I could not have accomplished all that I have.

My heart and soul is filled with gratitude

1

Chapter 1

Introduction to Adventure Cycling

I can remember when I was a kid in the late 60's learning how to ride my super cool bike. My dad bought me a Stingray style bike with the high rise handlebars, banana seat, and a funky, groovy color frame. Riding a bike came easy for me when dad took off the training wheels and gently guided me down the street, as he released his support allowing me to push the pedals into my new found freedom. To this very day, I still find a smile on my face and a subtle joy in my heart every time I go out and ride my bike.

So much so that in 2023 I rode my bike from Washington, DC to Eugene, OR on my first big bike adventure across the country. I chose to do it solo and self-contained, meaning I carried everything I needed on my bike.

The purpose of this short guide book is to share the key things to consider when planning your first bike adventure, whether it be one long weekend, a seven day tour, a month or even longer. My intention is to inspire more people to explore the great outdoors, traveling by bike. My hope is that you want to plan and go on a bike tour as soon as possible.

What is Adventure Cycling?

Adventure Cycling can be defined in different ways, but basically involves riding a bicycle over relatively long distances, experiencing different places and communities, and often camping overnight. The best thing about Adventure Cycling, Bike-packing, or Bike Touring is that it can be a relatively low cost way of getting some serious adventures into your life, if you like that sort of thing. Just you, your bike, maybe a companion or a small group, and the path that lies in front of you.

Because of this form of outdoor enjoyment, this pastime is quickly rising in popularity in recent years. Bicycle touring has been happening for many years; however, lots of people from all walks of life have become bored with their 9-5, their life in general, and want to "Get Out There" as my Adventure Cycling mentor Ryan Van Duzer would say.

Who Am I?

Just a little bit about myself, at the time I rode my bike across the country, I was 60 years young, in very good health, and was able to create the liberty and freedom I desired to do this adventure. I grew up as a Military Officer's brat traveling and moving a lot as a youngster. I was actively involved in sports in school having played basketball, a little football, and ultimately in High School, got into running on my school track team. Cross Country running was my favorite as I loved trail running and being in nature. After college, I moved to Vermont to work in the Alpine Ski Industry in Marketing and Sales. After six years of living in New England and falling in love with Mountain biking, I took a six week road trip and ski adventure with a buddy of mine out West to Colorado, Montana, and Utah. I quickly fell in love with the endless big blue skies, thin, dry air, and the overall lifestyle of being in the West that I decided to move to Colorado in 1993. I never looked back, and began to create my new life filled with skiing, hiking and cycling.

Unfortunately, I took my health for granted in my 40's, and I put most of the outdoor active hobbies I loved to do aside to begin a family life. In my early 50's my physical health had deteriorated to the point I was unable to enjoy a full day on the slopes, much less hike or bike any Colorado hill or mountain. I made a conscious choice to change that and begin the long, hard journey to regain my health and fitness. I also became very committed to my personal and spiritual growth in every area of my life. It took me almost 10 years of focused training and countless hours of personal and spiritual growth work to bring me to the point I was ready to tackle the thought of riding my bike across the country, but I did it!

Why Travel By Bicycle?

Bicycle travel isn't for everyone; however, almost everyone can ride a bike. I have seen people of all ages, all races, all genders, all income levels, and from all walks of life riding bicycles and enjoying Adventure Cycling. On my cross country bike trip, I met a woman who said she was 75 years old riding solo, self contained, from Seattle, WA to Jamestown, VA on the Trans America route. I met a young man pulling a bike trailer with his dog traveling with him. I met another woman who had never done a bike tour before, riding a $500 dollar Walmart Special bike carrying way too much gear in all the wrong places, traveling by bike. I ended up following her on Facebook and each post she made just amazed me that she was doing what she was, with no experience whatsoever. She actually completed her trip across the country in around 120 days, and did the whole thing with a big smile on her face. I met a couple from Germany that were riding bikes they picked up somewhere, but really had no business doing what they were doing; however, they sure seemed to be having a lot of fun doing what they loved to do together... Being free and enjoying their life to the fullest.

I wasn't 100% sure I would enjoy my trip because I was going to ride a very heavy bike for the first time, but what I found out was that I loved every moment of it. I actually love riding my loaded down bike; I love meeting people and going to new places, but most of all, I love being the master of my own destiny. Traveling by bike allowed me to slow down for once in my life, be in the present moment, while not necessarily knowing exactly where I was going to sleep that night, and sometimes, not even knowing where my next meal was coming from. And the coolest thing was that I was never disappointed. I met amazing people that were so kind and generous each and every day. In fact...I didn't meet one asshole during the entire 80 day bike tour.

Is Adventure Cycling for you?

I can't answer that, but if you enjoy the freedom of riding your bike, love being outdoors, meeting great people, and visiting beautiful places, Adventure Cycling may just be for you.

2

Chapter 2

Bicycle Safety and Responsible Etiquette:

- Wear a bicycle helmet
- Be sure your bicycle is in good operating condition. Recommend taking a class at your local bike shop or watch YouTube videos for basic bike maintenance and repairs. Carry a spare tube and tools for minor repairs. Practice changing a tire and lubricating your chain.
- Wear high visibility clothing.
- Bring proper clothing for all weather conditions. Layering is the best method. Light weight, breathable base layers and a two piece rain suit is highly recommended. I love Merino Wool socks and t-shirts, as they don't hold odors and can be worn many days before needing to be washed. Bringing proper clothes is critically important. It is no fun being cold, wet, and miserable on a bike tour. A whole book can be written on clothing and gear, but that is not the point of this book. Just do your research; watch YouTube videos about the best gear and clothing to bring, but know the more

comfortable you are on your tour, the more enjoyable the experience will be when weather conditions change for the worse, which they very likely will. Be prepared!

- Mount front and rear lights on your bike. Rechargeable lights work best. The rear red blinky light is the most important, and it is always suggested to have a front light, even if you only ride in the day. You never know when you might go through a tunnel, or get caught finishing your ride after dark.

- Have the ability to carry at least three to five liters of water. If you are camping, you might want to have a three liter water bag to fill when you get to a campground or have a trusted water source to provide the extra water needed when cooking and cleaning. Electrolytes are a must! Find out what works best for you, but I carried electrolyte tablets to add to my water bottle a couple of times each day.

- Carry a basic first aid kit. Take a first aid class if you are not familiar with basic first aid. Bad cycling accidents are rare, but minor scrapes and road rash from a slip or fall can happen. Be prepared!

- Keep your bicycle speed reasonable for safe bike control, and this may vary depending on your cycling ability, traffic and road conditions. Ride single file if on roads and with a group of people. Always allow at least one bike length between you and the person in front of you. Adjust your spacing as needed to allow motor vehicles to pass safely.

- I don't always do this, but it is best practice to comply with all applicable state and federal motor vehicle regulations when riding on roads. If you are on bike paths, the general rule and speed limit is 15 mph or less. That shouldn't be an issue for most riders who carry extra weight on their bike. I think I averaged around 10 - 12 mph on my trip across the country. Just stay in control of your bike, be mindful and kind to everyone on your route, and be cautious on down hills and gravel.

In short, a bike adventure is not a race. Take your time, enjoy the view; stop often to smell the flowers, take a picture, enjoy a snack break and meet someone interesting. Say hi to everyone, smile and be kind! That goes a long way to allowing the Law of Attraction to bring you all the good that life has to offer. That goes for on or off the bike.

3

Chapter 3

What kind of bike should I ride?

The short answer to this question is whatever bike you have! It is amazing to me to see people riding bikes for long distances using very inexpensive, sometimes old, but in good working condition bicycles. It is rarely about the bike that determines the success of a bike adventure. Sure, if the bike is falling apart as you ride, it will greatly diminish how much fun you will be experiencing. Amazingly, I have seen people on old, well maintained, heavy bikes having the time of their life. Basically, the lighter the bike, the more expensive it is going to be. No matter how expensive your bike is, it must be well maintained in order for it to work properly without something going wrong. I also highly recommend getting a professional bike fit for what every bike you choose to ride. This makes all the difference having a bike that fits you properly on those long days in the saddle. Most any bicycle shop can recommend a good bike fitter in your area.

Things to look for in a quality bike:

1. Quality tires that are not dry-rotting. Wheels that are true and not wobbling all over the place.

2. A well lubed chain that is not full of rust and wear. Most chains, if well maintained, will last between 1500 to 3000 miles. As with most of the components on any bike, chains come in a "Good, Better, and Best category. If you are doing long rides, I don't recommend cutting corners and buying a cheap chain, and the price difference is fairly marginal. It is never any fun when your chain breaks on a ride. It is generally a show stopper for many riders who don't know how to replace or repair a broken chain. (A short note on lubes: Use a high quality chain lube every 50 to 125 miles, depending on moisture, dust and dirt buildup.) Lubes come in Dry or Wet. Search on YouTube to learn what is best for you and your riding conditions, as well as how to apply.)

3. Bike cables are in good condition. Most cables should be replaced every 2500 to 5000 miles, depending on exposure and how they are used. If the cable casings are cracked and/or the ends are all frayed, replace them!

4. Good brakes! This is a must. Although I don't brake much when riding, I love having the ability to control my speed and stop when needed. Today, Disc brakes are all the rage and rightfully so. If maintained well, Disc brakes are the best brakes on the market; however, many older bikes have cantilever brakes of some sort, so always check the condition of your brake pads.

5. Front and rear Derailleur are in good working condition. If bent, replace them; If out of alignment, tune them.

6. If the bike has suspension of any kind, check to see it is in

good working condition and not in need of repair.

7. No stress fractures in your bike frame.

It is highly recommended to have a certified bike mechanic check your bike over to assure your bike is in good working condition. You can expect to pay anywhere from $75 to over $250 or more to get a quality tune up. In general, the more expensive your bike, the more expensive the tune will be. Hence why I love watching YouTube videos about bike tuning, and then doing some work myself to save money. Unfortunately, I am not a professional bike mechanic, so I certainly rely on them for any work I don't feel comfortable doing myself.

But I want to buy a new bike for my adventure...

Well, there are lots of choices today when buying your bike. I'm not a fan of "under biking" for something I plan to enjoy for long periods of time in the saddle. You know, buying the cheapest, simplest bike you can find. But, if that is your thing, so be it. Just don't be complaining when things go wrong, components keep breaking, and your easy day on the bike now becomes a long arduous endeavor. If I am looking to buy a new or slightly used bike, here are the things I would consider for my purchase.

1. What is my budget? Of course you can always find deals if you look hard enough; however, A new, decent bike today for long distance or adventure cycling will cost as little as $1200, and as much as $5000 or more. I don't recommend getting a very expensive, light weight, carbon or Titanium touring bike. It is just not necessary, because you are going to be carrying a bit of weight anyway. It is

way more important to have the proper gearing and quality components than a lightweight frame for bike touring. Most bikes used for touring are traditional steel frames or Aluminum. You should be able to find a quality bike anywhere from $1800 to $3500 pretty easily. I bought a new Surly Disc Trucker for around $2500, and I was overall, very happy with my choice.

2. Consider what kind of surfaces you will be riding? Will you be on all hard surface roads or will you be on some gravel trails, or even single track? Today there are several types of bikes that most people ride on Adventure Tours. Note: there are many different handlebar designs on the market today, but for this purpose, I am going to keep it simple using standard handlebar design. You can always upgrade to other handlebar designs if you choose.

3. Consider how much hill climbing you will be doing. Talk with a professional or watch YouTube videos to better understand gear ratios and what works best for hill climbing. I know I love having gears to choose from and quickly get to my "granny gear" when climbing hills. My bike has three chain rings in the front and 9 in the back with enough gear ratio to carry a heavy bike and me up steep hills and mountains. It makes all the difference in the world having the proper gears when needed.

4. Consider how you are going to carry all this gear. This is a big consideration and can be quite expensive. It all depends on how much gear you plan to carry. The more bags and space you have to carry your stuff, the more stuff you will bring. So, please put some thought into this consideration. I love my Ortlieb bags, and chose to have front and rear bags, along with a handlebar bag and top tube bag. My

bike and gear weighed close to 100 lbs by the time I loaded everything I needed to bring for a solo, self-contained bike tour. If your bike won't handle bike racks and the ability to carry panniers, consider attaching a bike trailer to your bike.

5. Consider what kind of bike tour you will be doing and how many days you will be traveling. Will you be needing to carry food and large amounts of gear and water? Will you be camping or staying in hotels? Below is a list of different styles of Adventure touring.

6. Un-assisted group tour. Riding with a small group to help share the load and weight of all the gear.

7. Assisted or supported group or individual tour. This means using a sagg or support vehicle to help carry gear and food.

8. Luxury, Inn to Inn style tours with full support (most of these tours are 5 to 10 days long) No need to carry any more gear than what you need for the day.

9. Solo, self-contained tour. Total freedom to do as short or as long as you like. This means you have to bring and pack everything you need to camp and feed yourself.

10. Racing styles tours, like the Great Divide Tour or Race Across America. (If you are doing these tours, you probably are not reading this book.)

Examples of different bikes that work well for bike touring

Drop-down handlebar road bike

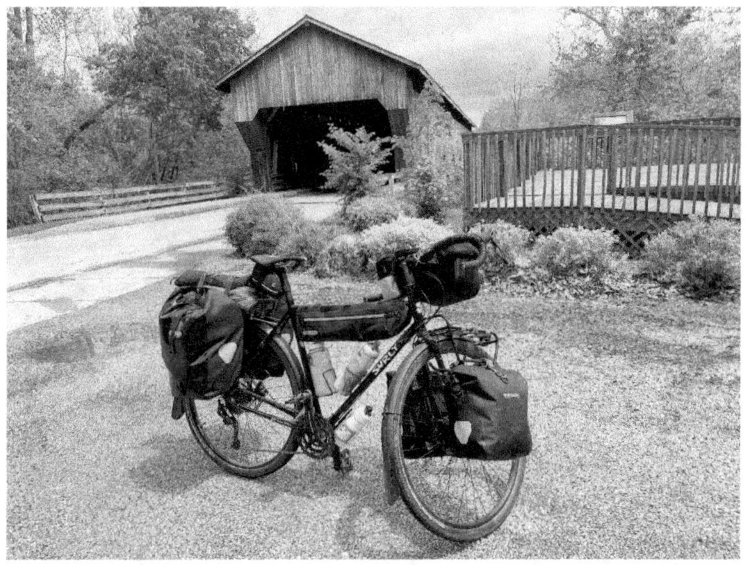

This photo is of my bike that I rode across the US. This is fully loaded with all my gear, food and water, and weighs about 100 lbs. I think the bike weighed 35 lbs, my gear weighed approximately 45 lbs, plus food and water. Not light by any means, but the gearing and geometry of the bike was designed for bike touring and carrying weight. It had tires I could ride on most any surface, and I thoroughly enjoyed building this bike designed specifically for Adventure Cycling.

Drop-down handlebar gravel bike

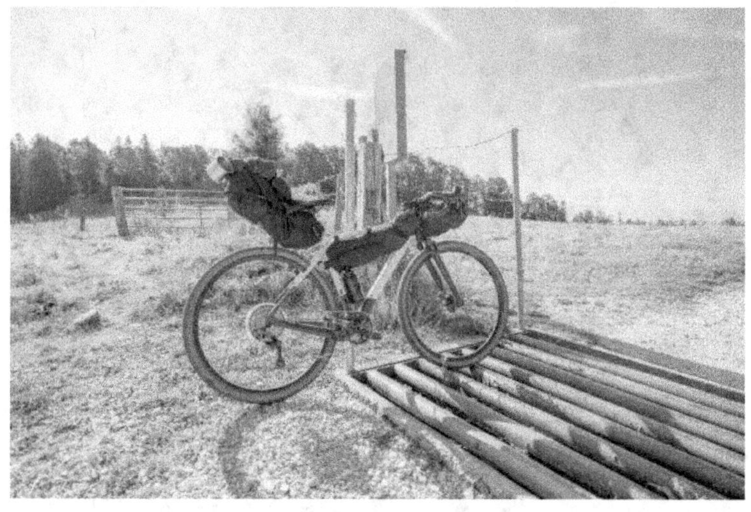

Gravel bikes are great for dirt roads and easy single and double track riding. Not all gravel bikes are designed for bike packing, but with all the new designs for strapping on bags today, this bike can work very well for a lot of people. This style bike is mostly used for bike packing off of hard surface roads. This might be intimidating for beginners.

Mountain bike (hard-tail with front suspension or no suspension at all) Best for Singletrack or rough, gravel routes.

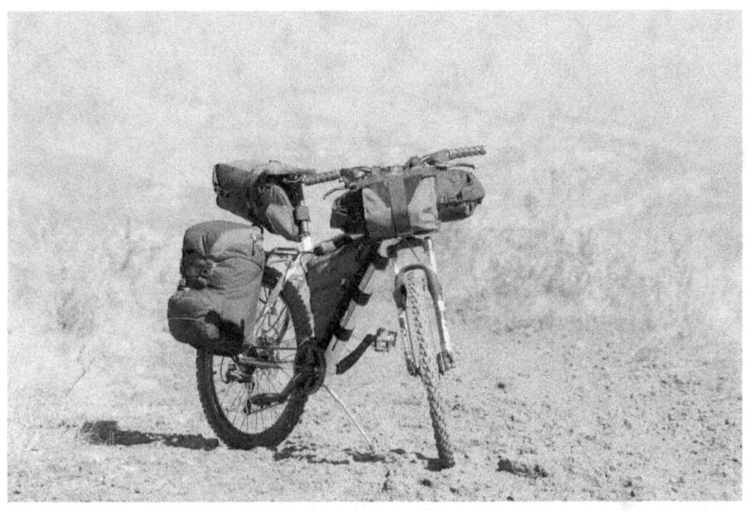

Most Mt. bikes have great gearing ratios for easier hill climbing and handle much better on rougher trails. Unfortunately, most Mt. bikes are not set up to install racks easily and the bike geometry isn't as comfortable for long, extended bike tours. There are a few on the market today. Priority Bicycles out of New York City has designed a good one for bike touring. I think Surly and Canyon have a couple, and of course Trek and Specialized Mt. bikes can be modified to work as well. The disadvantage of fatter tire bikes is that they don't ride as well on hard surfaces. Not a big deal if you ride solo, but if you are trying to keep up with others on road style bikes, this might be an issue to consider.

Gravel/road bike with trailer

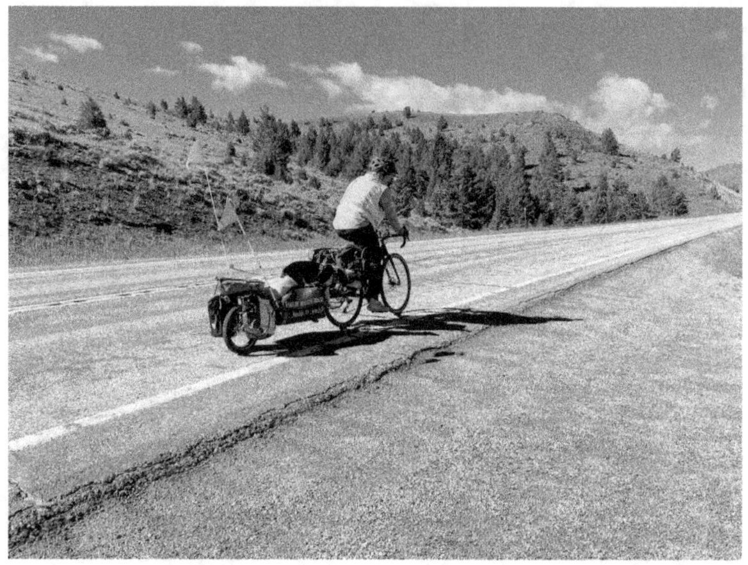

Trailers work great if your bike does not have the ability to install racks and strap on panniers or bike bags. They also work well if you are planning to carry your dog, as shown in this photo. I met and rode with this young man from Southern Colorado for a couple of weeks. He was a very strong guy but had very little bicycling experience prior to his Adventure Cycling tour. I think he rode from Pueblo, CO to Seattle, WA. No matter how hard the ride got, this dude kept a smile on his face and took on every challenge like a pro.

Electric Assist bikes

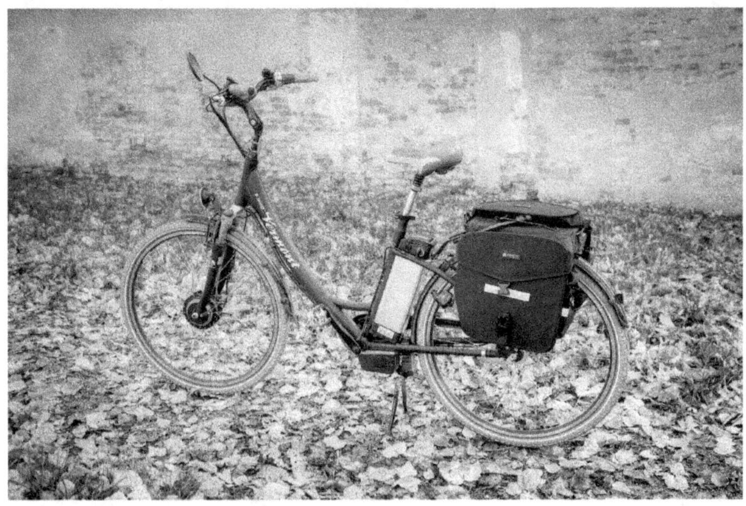

I love e-bikes, but I would not necessarily use them on a long distance bike tour. You may not always have an outlet available to plug-in and charge the bike when you need to. If you run out of power in the middle of your ride, you will be forced to peddle a very heavy bike with poor gears to choose from. Most people who purchase an e-bike are not necessarily in the best shape, so this may not be the best option for a long Adventure Tour. Where e-bikes work best is on supported bike tours. E-bikes allows anyone who rides them to keep up with others in your group. If the bike battery dies, you have support close by to help out. Although this is changing, e-bikes are generally better for day trips and not for long tours.

4

Chapter 4

Planning your Route

I want to be very clear that there is no right or wrong way to do a bicycle adventure. The most important thing is that you feel safe and have fun doing what you love. I cannot stress this enough, and wouldn't listen to anyone who tells you that you have to do it this way or that way. In fact, I saw as many ways to explore new places by bike as the many people I met doing it. So, with that in mind, let's jump into planning your big adventure.

I am a big fan of knowing my "WHY." In other words, why do I want to do this? Every person I have met who loves riding their bike, has a reason they do it. This mindset also has value when the times get tough, which they will, to keep moving forward. So, if you are not very clear on why you want to do adventure cycling, then I would highly suggest you take the time to do the inner mental work now before starting your bike adventure. If you are clear on your "why," then let's explore the options available.

Gratefully, there is a phenomenal resource available online called **Adventure Cycling Association**. Their website provides all the information anyone would need to enjoy Adventure Cycling. I would highly recommend using this extremely valuable resource when planning your bike adventure in the United States.

As I mentioned early, there is no right or wrong way to do this; however, thousands of people have completed amazing journeys on their bikes, so why not use their experience and wisdom to support what you want to do. Next to having a strong mindset, most everything else boils down to TIME and MONEY. So the next step is to figure out how much time you have and what is your budget to do what you want to do. Although I have met people doing this, I would not recommend jumping into a cross country ride as the first big adventure you undertake. This can be a bit overwhelming at first, so I would suggest taking smaller adventures, testing your set-up, and grow into the larger trips as things progress.

If you have the financial means to do a guided or supported bike tour, then this is a wonderful way to experience bike traveling. There are several bike tour companies in the US. By doing a simple search on the internet with a little research, I'm sure you can find a tour that works for you. I have used **Discovery Bike Tours** out of Vermont who lead Inn to Inn style tours all over the world. They pretty much do all the planning for you. All you have to do is book your flight to the starting location, and they take care of most everything else. Yeah, they can be a bit expensive; however, they can provide the bike, most meals, lodging, and sagg support services with at least two experienced guides to assure you safely get from point A to point B each day on the tour. There are less expensive options available, but as always... you get what you pay for. The cheaper the trip, the less amenities provided. If expensive bike tours are not your thing, then take some time to figure out what is. The point is just to get out there!

What route should I choose?

Basically, there are only four (4) types of routes available.

1. Road
2. Bike Path
3. Gravel roads and paths
4. Single and double track unpaved trails.

Unless you are an experienced cyclist and skilled mountain biker, I would not recommend Singletrack bike tours as your first option. For these involve a whole other set of skills and talents far above a beginner/novice level. And once again, I doubt you are reading this book if you are an advanced cyclist planning a big tour.

For your fist tour, I would recommend doing a **"Rails to Trails"** or bike path style tour. These are great because you can avoid roads and traffic. It allows you to be close to nature, play safe, and truly get into the experience of bicycle travel. There is an amazing non-profit organization called **"Rails to Trails Conservancy"** that has been involving communities all across the country to turn old Railroad Train Lines into bike and pedestrian paths. Their ultimate goal is to create a continuous bike path system from Washington, DC to Seattle Washington. They have a way to go to accomplish this lofty task; however, they are working hard, raising money, completing projects, and should make this happen in the next decade or so. Please consider financially supporting the Rails to Trails Conservancy, if you love cycling off roads as traffic flies by you.

I believe most every State in the US has created some type of bike path system, so check with your local bike shop, or search online, to find a bike path trail system near you. There are only a few trail systems that would be good for any overnight type experience. Many are fairly short, but there are a number of systems that are excellent for bike touring. Most are flat with little to know hills to climb as they tend to follow rivers or old train routes. My favorite is the **Katy Trail** which starts just North of St. Louis, MO and runs approximately 280 miles along the Missouri River towards Kansas City. I also love the **C&O Canal** from Washington, DC to Cumberland, MD, and from there, you can continue on the **Great Allegheny Passage or GAP Trail** from Cumberland, MD to Pittsburgh, PA. As I already said, most every State in the US has wonderful trail systems in place ready for you to explore. If your state doesn't have a good bike trial system, MOVE!

It does take a bit of planning for multi-day bike tours. I would say it takes at least one hour for every day you plan to ride. I know I spent over 6 months planning and preparing for my big tour across the country. And, that does not include training time. The first trip is always the most challenging, and of course, the planning gets a bit easier after doing this a few times.

Adventure Cycling Association is, by far, the best resource available to support most any US tour you want to do. It almost takes some of the fun out of planning because they have already done all the leg-work, know all the good places to stop for food, where to find water and food, bike shops, lodging, camping etc... They have wonderful cycling guide maps available to purchase, or you can download the routes on your bike computer. I love the printed maps because all the information you need is on them.

Where do I sleep when bike touring?

Well, that all depends on what kind of tour or adventure you want to experience. It also depends on what you enjoy doing and what your budget will allow. It can get pretty expensive if you stay in hotels/motels each night, but for a lot of people, that is what they prefer. Some call that a credit card tour, but this method can be more affordable if you are only traveling for a few nights. If you are planning a longer trip, you may want to consider camping when possible; however, that means having to pack and haul camping gear. I prefer camping as much as possible, only staying in a bed with a roof over my head when the weather is bad or there just isn't any other option. I had the setup to carry all my camping gear, and I am an experienced backpacker and an avid outdoor enthusiast. . I had most of my gear that I needed designed for lightweight camping, including a small, lightweight tent and sleeping bag, kitchen setup, and all the basic survival things needed to enjoy my camping experience.

Obviously, camping isn't for everyone, so another awesome option is using a cycling app called **Warm Showers**, which is staying at people's houses. When I did my ride across the US, it took me 80 days to complete my journey. I camped out for about 25 days, stayed in cheap motels or B&B type places for around 20 nights. I stayed at friends houses for about 7 nights, and the rest of the nights I stayed at Warm Shower host sites. With little exception, Warm Shower stays were one of the best experiences of my tour. I love Warm Showers! All the hosts were cyclists themselves and generally provided a comfortable bed, of course a warm shower, often a good meal or two, laundry services, bike tuning and great conversation. I met the most interesting people and loved every place I stayed. There are a couple of thousand

Warm Showers host locations across the country and many more in Europe. The App costs around $30 for the year, and is kind of like "a pay it forward" style thing. Meaning when you are not on a bike tour or out of town for whatever reason, they hope you will make your home available for other Adventure Cyclists to be a guest at your place. I have now had several bike-packers stay with me, and love meeting these very cool and interesting people. I highly recommend this App, but, unfortunately, there isn't always a host available when you want them.

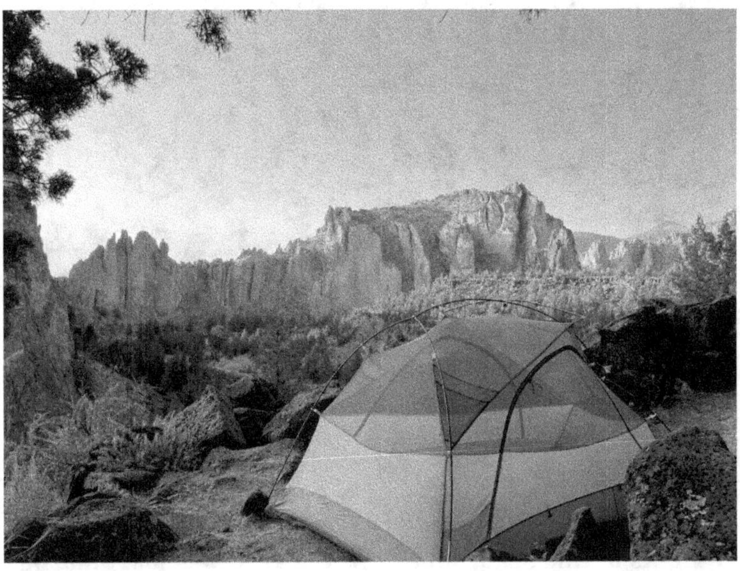

Hard to beat this camping spot at Smith Rock State Park in Oregon. I love camping, and when I can find beautiful places like this, it makes life on the trail even better! To me, camping is the way to go! Nothing beats being fully self-supported, preparing my own meals, and being open to receive all the goodness living in the outdoors provides. Yeah, it can be a bit tough when the weather turns for the worst, but this only makes you tougher, and allows you to better appreciate all that you have when back at home in your comfortable bed, hot shower, and full kitchen.

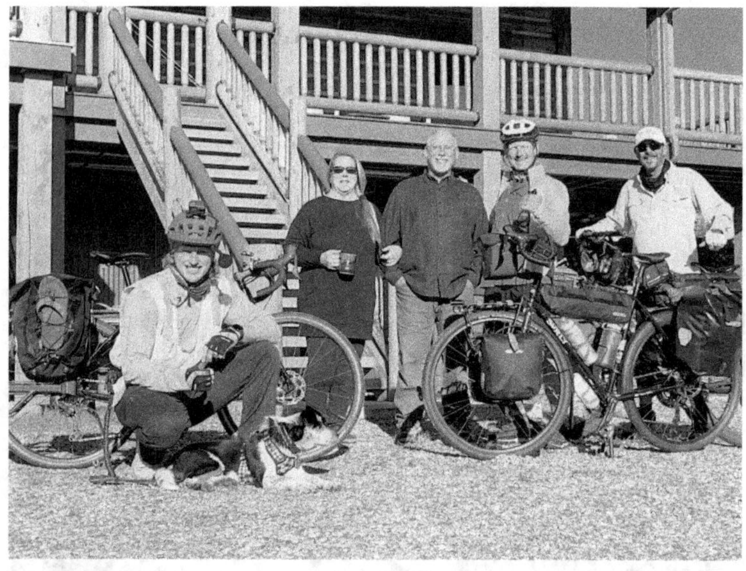

Incredible Warm Showers host in Innis, MT. I stayed a couple of nights at this beautiful ranch. Our host was just amazing, providing a very comfortable bed, great food, and wonderful conversation. I cannot say enough good things about Warm

Showers as it was a major highlight of my bike tour.

25

5

Chapter 5

Training and Mental Preparation

Cycling for long distances takes endurance and a certain level of physical fitness and a strong mental attitude. I do not recommend beginning a multi-day cycling trip without doing the necessary preparation to get your body and mind ready for the many challenges ahead. It takes a lot of fun away from your trip if your body is aching and your muscles are too sore to ride. The biggest complaint I hear from newbie cyclists is that their butt hurts so much that they cannot sit on the seat. It generally takes at least three to four weeks of regular cycling (that means 3-4 times a week) to get your butt muscles used to being in the saddle for an extended period of time. Bottom line.... Have several hundred miles completed or several months of training before starting any type of bike tour. You won't regret it!

Now, A lot depends on how much elevation, or climbing, your chosen route has, that will dictate how much physical training you will want to do. Hence, why I recommend starting on an easier, flatter route for your first bike adventure. Climbing hills is a skill and it takes practice to get more comfortable climbing them. I have been cycling for decades, train on almost a daily basis, and I spent 6 months of focused strength and endurance training before I started my ride across the country. And even with that level of physical preparation, I found that my body was not prepared to be in the saddle for six to eight hours a day. It is very difficult to train for that, but doing all the training I did, made all the difference in gradually becoming accustomed to life on a bike.

Most people who get into Adventure Cycling, bike-packing, or bike touring, get into it because they love to ride their bike, so I am going to assume that you already ride often and have some basic level of physical fitness. A lot also depends on our age and your general health. Please consult with a physician before doing any sort of extreme activities. Ideally, set your ego aside and assess your overall health to determine how much training you will want to do before attempting a long, hard ride on your bike.

I am not a big fan of gyms and pumping iron; however, strength training is a must do if you want to get stronger and have more power in your pedal stroke. I highly recommend a focus on core strength. This is because when your legs get tired, your core will kick in to help you finish a long, hard ride. I also suggest doing two or three times per week a series of deadlifts and squats using weights. Start with light weights and gradually increase the weight as you progress over time. Lunges, climbing stairs, box jumps or step-ups are very good as well, but be careful with your knees at all times. Once again, start easy and work your way up as you slowly get stronger over time.

If you are not familiar with how to do strength training, I strongly suggest you get with a PT (Physical Trainer) to coach you on how to safely perform these strengthening activities.

Every gym I have ever been in has trainers who would love to support and coach you to become stronger, better preparing you for the more challenging rides ahead. YouTube also has some very good videos to show you proper technique, but don't offer the needed feedback or coaching to check your form for safe strength training. If you want to get stronger safely, you will want to do strength training in the gym with some form of coaching and accountability.

Flexibility is also very important for cycling. I practice Yoga and perform general stretching on a daily basis. I find that stretching and flexibility training helps me minimize the risk of injury during workouts, as well as it is very calming. In Yoga, there is a strong element of breath work involved. Being mindful of your breath is very helpful when cycling, particularly on uphill climbs. I also have a daily meditation practice that has a focus on breath work, mindfulness, affirming my success and joy in everything inside and out. Having a strong mental attitude will carry you a long way when the body gets tired, the weather turns nasty, and Life throws those tough punches. I am sure we have all experienced it, but it is how we deal and think about those challenges that will make or break a person when the times get tough.

In conclusion, Adventure Cycling can be the best experience of your life; I know it is for me. There is nothing better than being in nature, being prepared for whatever comes your way, and riding my bike to experience amazing places and meeting beautiful people. It certainly isn't for everyone, but for those who love outdoor adventure, it is without a doubt, hard to beat. So, get out there and Love Life on a Bike!

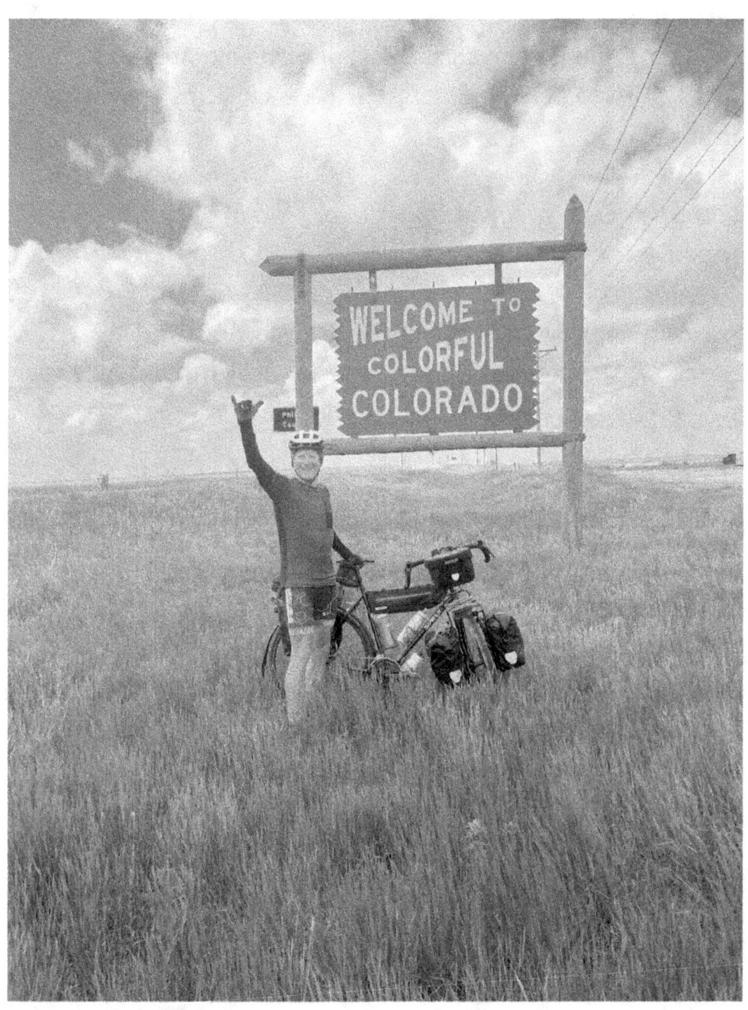

I hope you enjoyed this brief guide book about Adventure Cycling and Bike Touring, and feel inspired to prepare for your first adventure!

Resources

Rails to Trails Conservancy: Building a nation connected by trails. (2024, April 9). Rails to Trails Conservancy. https://www.railst otrails.org/

Warmshowers – a global community of touring cyclists. (n.d.). https://www.warmshowers.org/

Discover what awaits | Adventure Cycling Association. (2024, March 1). Adventure Cycling Association. https://www.adve nturecycling.org/

Ryan Van Duzertv host. (n.d.). Ryan Van Duzer. https://www.duz ertv.com/

Inn-to-Inn Bike Tours – Discovery Bicycle Tours. (n.d.). https://w ww.discoverybicycletours.com/

Waite Endurance. (2023, November 8). *Waite Endurance – Waite endurance.* https://www.waiteendurance.com/

The Fast Lab. (2024, February 3). *Sports Performance Training & Testing Lab Serving Denver, CO.* The FAST Lab. https://www.thef astlab.com/

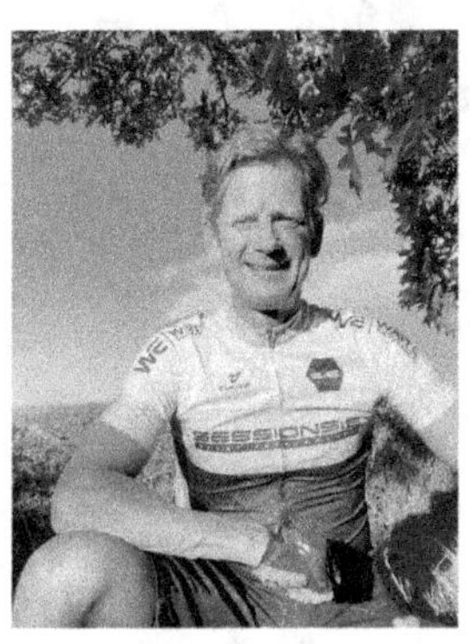

About the Author

Loving Life is my motto for just about everything I do. I am a believer that if I don't enjoy what I am doing, than I won't do it! I have dedicated myself to learning and growing in every area of my life ever since I took my first personal growth course in 1998. That was a benchmark for me, and I am forever grateful for all the seminars, courses, workshops, books and lectures I have participated in over the years. I have lived the last 28 years in the Denver Metro area of Colorado and currently reside in Chesapeake, VA, allowing me to be close to my father and special needs brother. I am an avid cyclist and outdoor enthusiast, carrying in my heart a deep appreciation for the world around me. I am so blessed to live the life of my dreams and grateful for the many friends and family that have made all this possible.

www.ingramcontent.com/pod-product-compliance
Lightning Source LLC
Chambersburg PA
CBHW051900250726
48659CB00006B/2321